To Air Is Human

A manual for people with chronic lung disease (COPD)

Researched and written by:

Madeline H. Barrow, B.S., M.Ed.
Nancy R. Hull, B.A.

Consultants:

Jill Malen, R.N., M.S., N.S.
Robert M. Bruce, M.D., FACP
Sally Crim Tibbals, R.N., B.S.N.
                        M.S., PCNS

This book should not replace the advice or treatment
your doctor gives you. It is to add to what you are
already learning about chronic lung disease.

Authors:

Madeline H. Barrow, B.S., M.Ed, is a professional writer residing in the metro Atlanta area. She provided much of the original research for the book.

Nancy R. Hull, B.A., served as an author and editor. She is co-owner of Pritchett & Hull.

Consultants:

Jill Malen, R.N., M.S., N.S.
Pulmonary Clinical Nurse Specialist
Barnes Hospital
St. Louis, MO

Robert M. Bruce, M.D., FACP
Pulmonary Disease Specialist
Barnes Hospital
St. Louis, MO

Sally Crim Tibbals, R.N., B.S.N., M.S., PCNS
Professor of Nursing
Oklahoma City Community College
Oklahoma City, OK

Reviewer:

Ralph L. Haynes, M.D.
Director, Steiner Lung Center
St. Joseph's Hospital
Atlanta, GA

And a special thanks to **John E. Huffman, B.A., CRTT**, who worked with us early in the development of this book and to **Becky Fitzgerald,** Assistant Director of Pulmonary Rehab at Emory University Hospital.

Design, Illustrations: **Michèle Williams**
Editing: **Faye Hoffman**
Pritchett & Hull Associates, Inc.
Title: **Anthony Williams**

What's In This Book

A Word About COPD

COPD stands for chronic obstructive pulmonary disease. Chronic means long-term. Obstructive refers to blockage in the airways of the lung. Pulmonary refers to the lungs.

The most common lung diseases are:

- chronic bronchitis

- emphysema

- asthma

- bronchiectasis

- cystic fibrosis (CF)

The main symptoms are shortness of breath, coughing, wheezing or too much mucus in the lungs. You may have one or more of these symptoms.

Living with chronic lung disease means learning to control it, and the best way to control your disease is to be an active partner in your treatment. Practice daily what you learn from this book. Ask your doctors any questions you may have. Then, when breathing problems or infections occur, you will know just what to do. You will be in control and feel good about yourself.

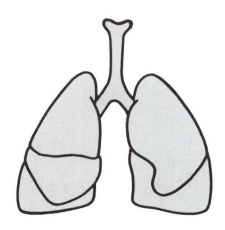

Chapter 1

Practice
Practice
Practice

Water drinking

A most important treatment for lung disease is to drink a lot of water or other fluids each day. Fluids keep mucus thin so that it can be coughed up and out.

A buildup of thick, sticky mucus in the lungs is a main cause of shortness of breath, wheezing or dry, hacking coughs. Thick mucus is also a breeding ground for infection.

It may take a few days to a week or so of drinking a lot of fluids to notice a change in mucus. For most people this means drinking 2 to 4 quarts of water and other fluids a day.* This much fluid will make you urinate more, but, in time, your body will adjust.

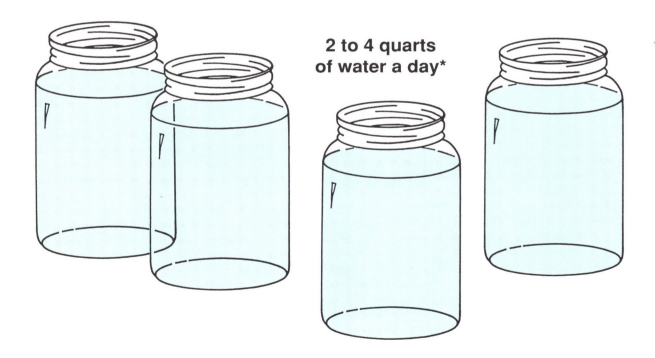

2 to 4 quarts of water a day*

* Ask your doctor if 2 to 4 quarts of fluid a day is OK for you. **Some people can't drink a lot of fluids** because of kidney disease, prostate trouble or heart disease.

You can drink juice as part of your 2 to 4 quarts, but count calories if you are trying to lose or gain weight. To keep from feeling bloated, don't drink more than 1 to 2 glasses of fluid per hour, and don't drink a lot close to mealtime.

Don't drink a lot of colas, tea or coffee with caffeine. These make the body lose water and can cause you to feel nervous and "jittery." Small amounts of drinks with caffeine are OK — 2 to 4 cups a day. Some people with asthma find coffee helps relieve wheezing at times.

Don't use antihistamines, diuretics ("water pills") or cough suppressants unless your doctor tells you to take them for some other problem. These drugs dry the body out and make mucus thicker. **Water is the best expectorant.** Expectorants, other than water or other liquids, are rarely prescribed for someone with chronic lung disease.

Controlled coughing

When mucus is thin, do this:

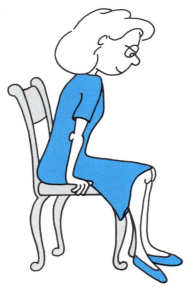

1. Sit up and lean your head forward slightly.

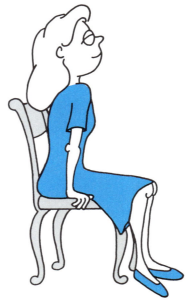

2. Take a deep, slow breath through your nose, and hold it for 2 seconds.

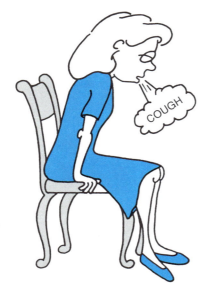

3. Cough once (to loosen mucus).

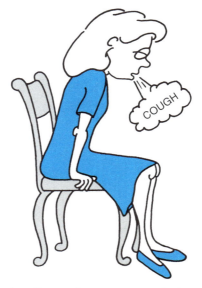

4. Cough a second time (to move mucus forward).

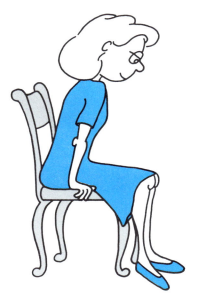

5. Wait a few seconds.

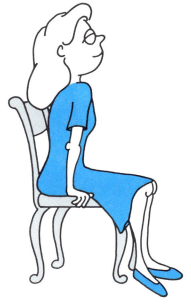

6. Sniff gently to inhale. (If you take a big breath, it may push the mucus back into the lungs and make you cough again.)

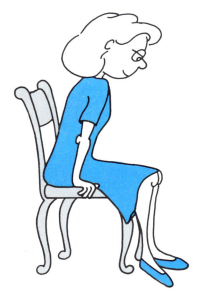

7. Relax.

Repeat these steps if you still need to cough.

This is called **"controlled coughing."** It works when the mucus in your lungs has been thinned by lots of fluids. (Keep on drinking 2 to 4 quarts of fluid each day if allowed.)

Do controlled coughing with small, short coughs. Avoid large blasts of air.

You need to cough up mucus when you can. Coughing is one of nature's ways of cleaning the lungs. Each day your lungs make extra mucus in response to "dirt" from smoke, pollution or germs you may inhale. If you don't get rid of this extra mucus, you increase your chances of having shortness of breath, wheezing, infections or plugged airways.

Don't waste energy trying to cough up thick mucus. This will irritate the lungs and do little to help your breathing problem. A long coughing spell can wear you out. This is why controlled coughing, after mucus is thin, is best. It is the easiest way to rid your lungs of excess mucus.

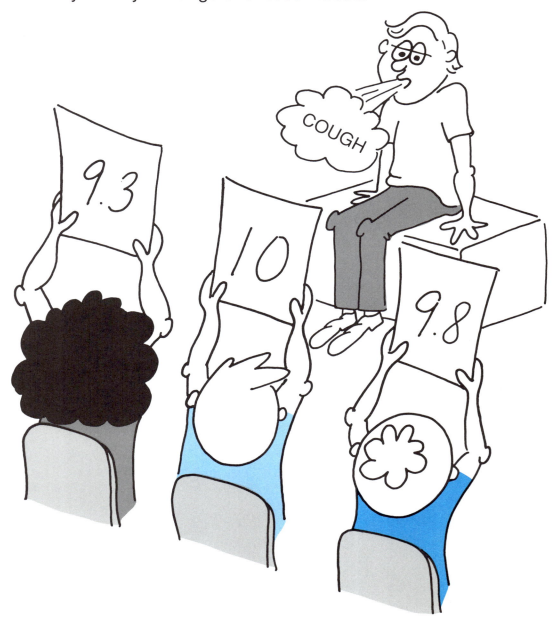

Pursed lips breathing

Pursed lips breathing works when you find it hard to breathe. Learn this now so you won't panic when you feel short of breath.

1. Breathe in slowly through your nose for 2 counts.

2. Purse your lips as if you were going to whistle.

3. Breathe out gently through pursed lips for 4 slow counts. (Exhale twice as slowly as you inhale.) Let the air escape naturally. Do not force the air out of your lungs.

4. Keep doing pursed lips breathing until you are not short of breath.

This way of breathing slowly can be done anywhere at any time.

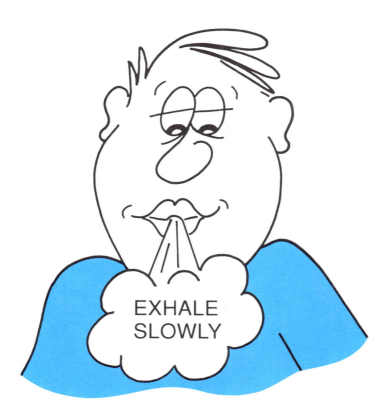

EXHALE
SLOWLY

Pursed lips breathing helps trapped, stale air get out of your lungs. When you have COPD, your lungs are better at taking air in than letting air out. Stale air gets trapped in your lungs, keeping fresh air out. When this happens, you feel tightness in the chest or short of breath. Breathing faster will not bring you relief. Breathing out slowly through pursed lips will.

Practice pursed lips breathing every day. Don't wait until you are in a breathing crisis to learn how to breathe more slowly. You may be too panicked to believe something as simple as pursed lips breathing can help.

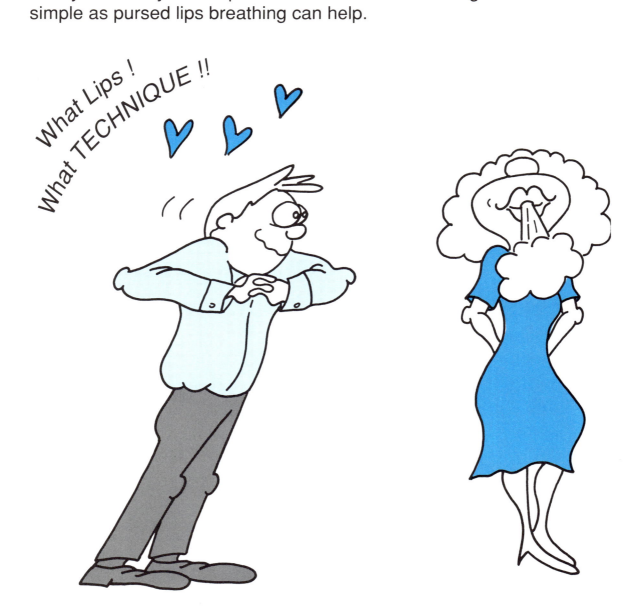

Checklist for Chapter 1

Check off the things you have learned and are now using in your daily care.

- [ ] I drink 2 to 4 quarts of water and other fluids each day.
- [ ] I can do controlled coughing.
- [ ] I can do pursed lips breathing when I feel short of breath.

Things to remember:

- Ask your doctor the right amount of liquid for you to drink each day. (Some people can't drink a lot of fluid because of other medical problems.)

- Avoid too much caffeine. It makes the body lose fluid.

- Water is the best expectorant.

- Do controlled coughing when mucus is thin.

- Practice pursed lips breathing every day so you can use it when you need it.

- If you are not sure you are doing controlled coughing or pursed lips breathing the right way, get your doctor, nurse or therapist to help you.

Notes _____

_____

_____

_____

_____

_____

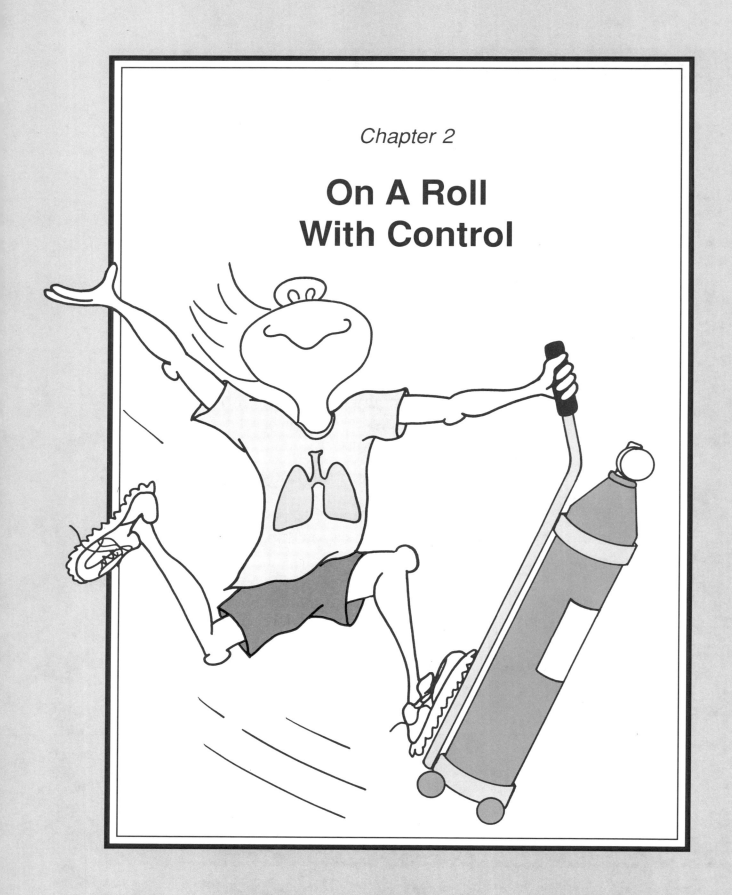

Chapter 2

On A Roll
With Control

Here are some of the problems and treatments you will deal with as you control your lung disease.

When you are wheezing

1. Do **pursed lips breathing** (pp. 11-12). As you gently exhale against pursed lips, the airways stay open, and air flows out more easily.

2. Take your **prescribed bronchodilator.** Bronchodilators relax the muscles around the airways so they open up.

3. **Keep drinking fluids -** 2 to 4 quarts a day (if allowed).

Wheezing is the noise you hear when exhaled air whistles through partly blocked air tubes (bronchi). You may wheeze because the muscles around these tubes squeeze in when something irritates them (asthma). Or you may wheeze when you have too much mucus in your airways (bronchitis). Sometimes people with emphysema wheeze because the small airways in the lungs have collapsed. And if your **body tends to "hold water,"** the lining of your airways may swell, causing wheezing.

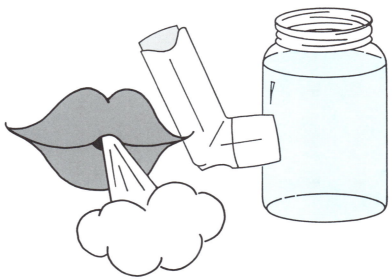

When you have too much mucus or infection

Drink 2 to 4 quarts of fluid a day (if allowed), and do controlled coughing (pp. 8-10) to bring up mucus. When mucus pools in the lungs too long, it gets thick and sticky and can become infected.

When you are able to cough up mucus, check the color. Healthy mucus is white, clear and watery. Infected mucus is yellow, brown, green or streaked with blood. If your mucus is colored or contains blood, call your doctor. He or she may prescribe an antibiotic for the infection. If an antibiotic is prescribed, take every dose so the medicine can get rid of all the infection.

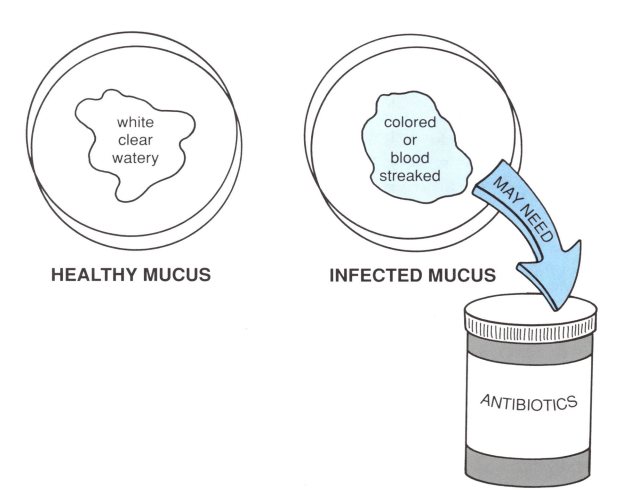

white
clear
watery

HEALTHY MUCUS

colored
or
blood
streaked

INFECTED MUCUS

MAY NEED

ANTIBIOTICS

Smoking

If you smoke, find some way to quit. Emphysema and chronic bronchitis are diseases of smokers. No matter how long you have smoked, stopping now will help you breathe better. Many carcinogens (agents that cause normal cells to change to cancerous cells) have been found in cigarette smoke.

If you stop smoking, you can slow down the serious damage you are doing to yourself. With every puff, a smoker irritates and damages the lining of the lungs. Mucus builds up, the airways swell and the membranes through which oxygen and carbon dioxide are exchanged are destroyed. Then the heart must work harder to pump more blood because the body is crying out for more oxygen.

Try not to breathe in anyone else's smoke either. This is called passive smoking, and it can harm your lungs, too.

Call your hospital, lung association, clinic or public health nurse to see if there is a stop smoking or other support group to help you quit. Ask your doctor about Nicorette gum. It has helped a lot of people stop smoking (most often when the people also attended support group meetings).

Many people have to try to stop smoking more than once before they succeed. So don't give up! Keep trying, and you will win the battle with the smoking habit.

Air outside and inside

Pollution

In places where the air is polluted, more people have chronic bronchitis and emphysema. If you can, stay inside a centrally heated or air-conditioned building on days when the pollution count is high (100 or above).* Always avoid being exposed to air pollution when you can.

Keep your heating and air-conditioning system in good working order. Change filters often.

Weather

Breathing in very cold air can make you cough and wheeze. Breathe through a handkerchief or scarf to warm the air before it hits your lungs. **You can now buy cold weather masks** as well.

Either a humid or dry climate can be a problem. An **air-conditioner or a dehumidifier** can dry out air that is too damp. A humidifier can be used to moisten air that is too dry. (Dry air is often a problem in winter when the heat is on.) A humidifier can also be used to settle dust. **Clean all humidifiers often.**

You may have to try it out to see whether a damp or dry climate suits you best. A humidity of 40 to 50% is most often the best for easy breathing.

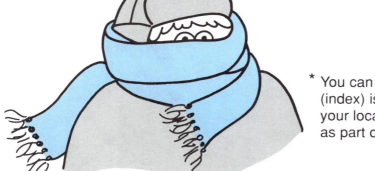

* You can usually find what the pollution count (index) is by calling weather information at your local TV station. Often this count is given as part of the weather update on the news.

18

Household fumes

Avoid strong fumes from cleaning products, and use a venting fan over the stove to get rid of cooking fumes. Use products which are poured or rubbed instead of those sold in spray cans. Sprayed fumes are easy to inhale.

Dust

Dust-raising jobs in your house or yard can make it harder for you to breathe. If you must do a "dusty" job, wear a handkerchief, dust mask or filter over your mouth and nose. Best of all, have someone else dust your house when you aren't home. Stay away from your house for at least 45 minutes after it has been cleaned and dusted.

Allergies

If you know you are **allergic** to something (such as cats, dogs, grass, trees), stay away from it as much as you can. Sleep in a room cooled by an **air-conditioner with a CLEAN filter** instead of in a room cooled by a window fan. Fans draw in mold and pollen. Dirty air filters attract mold and germs. Your doctor will suggest medicine or allergy shots if you need them.

Your emotions

Mood changes can affect how well you breathe. Your emotions can cause the muscles used for breathing to tighten, making airways narrow and breathing hard. And when you feel bad, you don't take good care of yourself.

Learning to deal with all kinds of moods will be important to how well you breathe. Lung disease is not fun, and daily treatment can be a real bore. Having someone to talk to helps a lot. Don't try to keep your feelings to yourself. No one can help you if you do. Walking and relaxation or breathing exercises may help a lot. If you stay in pain or are depressed for weeks, no matter what you try, talk with your doctor. He or she can help you get back on track and breathing more freely.

Here are some of the moods you may have at one time or another.

Shock and disbelief

Some people can't believe they have a chronic disease. They may pretend for awhile that the disease doesn't exist. The best cure for this "shock" is time and understanding. Long talks with your family, doctor, nurses and therapists can help a lot.

Anger

Anger is a common response. It is OK to be mad, but don't take it out on yourself or others. Being open and direct with others will get the best results.

Find out why you are angry. Some people get mad when they have to accept help from others. Some are angry because of the changes in their daily lives caused by their lung disease. Once the real reason for anger is found, it is less harmful. Again, talk it out with your family, friends, doctor and therapist.

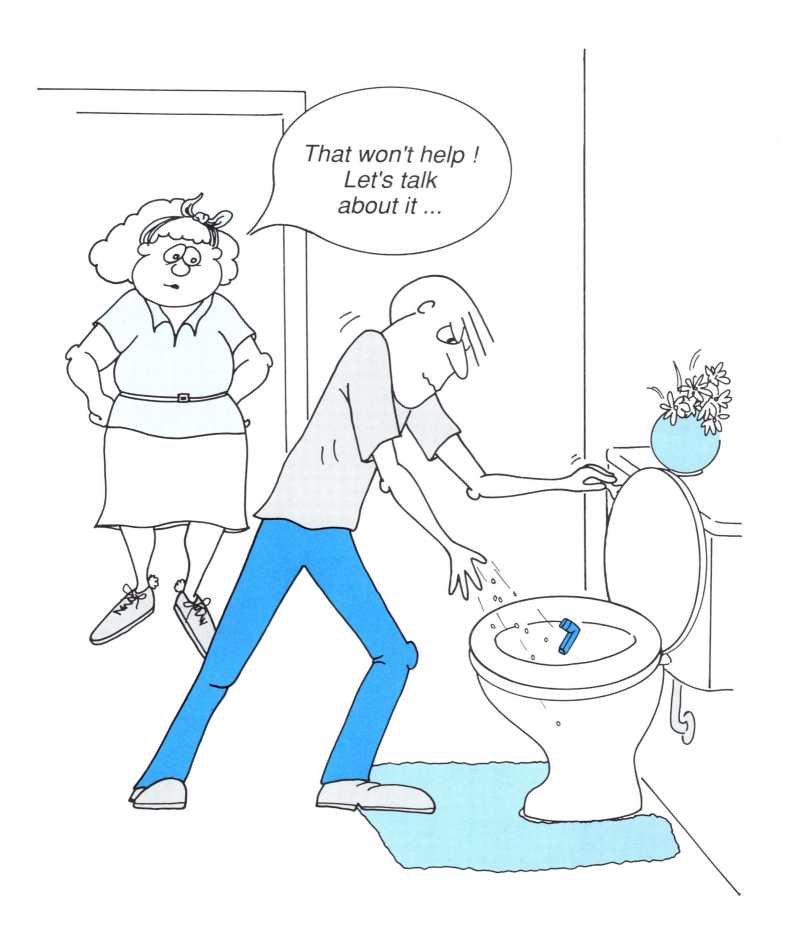

Sadness/depression

Sadness or depression often occurs when anger is turned inward toward one's self. Feelings of guilt are common, too. Sadness that goes on for a long time can be very painful and harmful. If this is true for you, let your doctor know. It can be treated. Some signs of depression are:

- changes in eating habits
- changes in sleep patterns
- withdrawal from family and friends
- loss of interest in daily activities

Some things that can help are keeping active, going to support groups, exercising and talking with your doctor or therapist.

Anxiety/fear

Fear is a normal response to shortness of breath, but fear can also make breathing harder. There are many ways to reduce fear or anxiety. Some are:

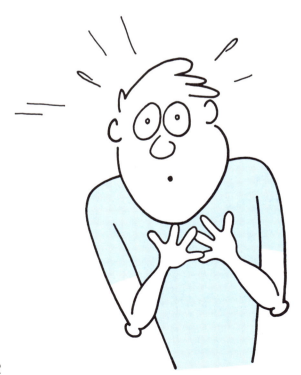

- identify the fear
- talk out your fear with others
- use pursed lips breathing
- practice relaxation exercises each day (see p. 24)
- rest some and exercise some each day

Acceptance/control

It takes practice to fit treatment into your daily routine. And at times you may feel less in control of your breathing than at others. Don't give up. No one likes having a chronic lung disease, but most accept it better when they learn to control the way they feel. As you adjust to your treatment, your sense of well-being will grow. You will control your lung disease rather than letting it control you.

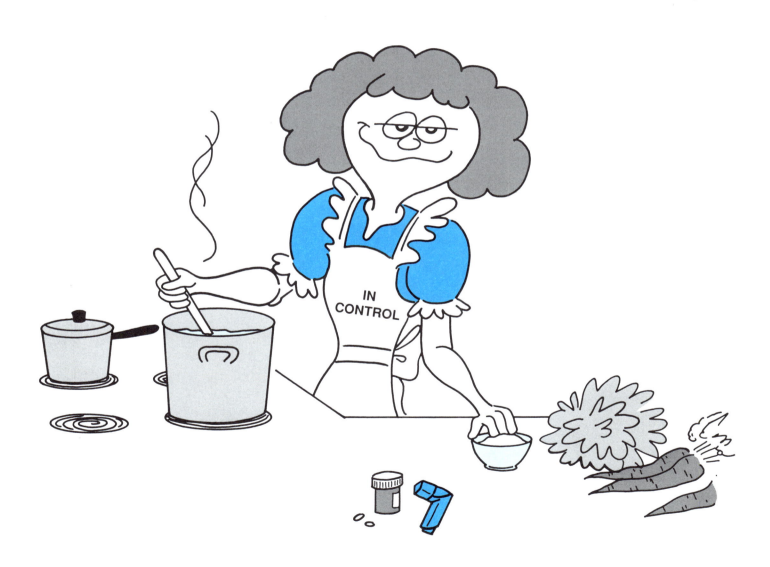

Relaxation exercises

When you relax your body and mind, you reduce muscle tension and relieve anxiety. Use these relaxation steps to relieve tension when breathing problems increase.

First, find a quiet, peaceful place. Lie down, and put a pillow under your head and knees, or sit up in a straight-backed armchair.

1. **Head and neck**
   Pull chin down towards chest as tightly as you can. Then push back of head into pillow. Turn head from side to side in a relaxed way. Let it stop when it comes to a comfortable position.

2. **Shoulders**
   Shrug shoulders and tighten shoulder muscles as much as you can, then let go.

3. **Arms** (Do one hand and one arm at a time.)
   Bend elbow and make a fist out of your hand. Tighten fist, then let go. Straighten arm and fingers. Tighten as much as you can, then let go.

4. **Legs** (Do one leg at a time.)
   Hold leg straight and point toe. Tighten leg muscles, then let go. Point toes toward your nose and push heel and back of leg into bed. Tighten, then let go.

5. **Back**
   Arch your back up like a cat. Tighten as much as you can, then let go. Do not lift your hips while arching.

6. **Face**
   Tighten ("scrinch") up all of your face muscles. Hold, then let go.

7. **Eyes**
   Focus your eyes on something. Watch it, and slowly let your eyelids grow heavy. Open your eyes, and then let them close slowly until they feel comfortable closed.

Medications

The list which follows has on it most of the drugs prescribed for lung disease. **Learn which drugs you take, what they are for and their side effects.** Tell your doctor if you feel these side effects at any time. Also, if you are taking more than one drug, your druggist can keep a list of them for you. Sometimes two or more drugs will interact and cause problems. Tell your doctor all of the drugs you are taking. Include those drugs ordered by other doctors and any over-the-counter drugs (even eye drops).

Carry a list of your medications in your purse or wallet. If you are in an emergency, this list can be very helpful to the doctor treating you.

If an inhaler medication is prescribed for you, be sure you know how to **use the inhaler properly.** Have your doctor, nurse or therapist show you how to use the inhaler. Have them watch you use it to see if you are doing it right.

CAUTION:

Do not take any of the drugs described in this section unless prescribed by your doctor.

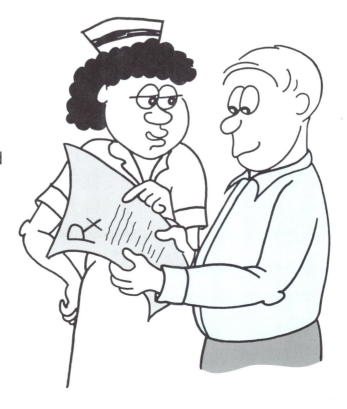

Bronchodilators

These drugs relax the muscles around the bronchial tubes. The tubes open up, and you breathe easier. Bronchodilators can be taken by pills, shots, liquids, aerosol sprays and suppositories (rarely).

Use bronchodilators only as your doctor tells you.
Take the amount prescribed at the times he or she tells you. If this medicine upsets your stomach, take it with food. Call your doctor if any of these possible side effects occur:

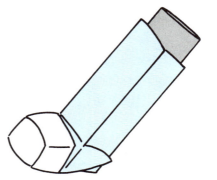

- irregular heartbeat

- nervousness

- restlessness

- trembling

- bad taste in mouth

- headache

- trouble sleeping

- nausea/vomiting or stomach pain

- more frequent urination
  (Most often happens when you first start taking drug. This decreases after awhile.)

Xanthines
- Take doses at evenly divided times during the day. (Example: twice a day - take every 12 hours)

- Do not take on an empty stomach.

- Avoid **large** amounts of coffee, tea or sodas with caffeine.

- Do not chew tablets.

- Do not take more medicine than your doctor has directed.

Beta stimulants (inhalers)

- Be sure you know how to properly use the inhaler.

- A spacer may also be prescribed. (See p. 33.)

- Use only amount your doctor tells you and only as often as directed.

- If you are using more than one puff for your dose, wait a few minutes between puffs.

- Store the inhaler away from heat and direct sunlight.

Beta stimulants (oral)

- Take only the dose your doctor prescribes.

- Do not take this drug more often than directed.

Parasympathetic blocker inhalers

- Know how to use the inhaler.

- If using more than one puff for a dose, wait a few minutes between puffs.

- Usual dose is 2 puffs, 3 times a day. You may use more puffs if needed, but the total number of puffs in 24 hours should not be more than 12. (Your doctor will tell you how many to use.)

- Do not store above 86° F (30° C); avoid a lot of humidity.

I take:

name:_____

dose:_____

time:_____

Steroids

Steroid drugs act in two ways. They decrease swelling of the airways and lungs and open (dilate) bronchial tubes. **Never change your dosage or stop taking steroids without your doctor's advice.** Steroids come in the same forms as bronchodilators (pills, shots, liquids, aerosol sprays).

Always take these pills with food, milk or an antacid liquid. If your stomach is still upset or you have pain or burning, call your doctor. Stomach problems are more likely to occur if you drink alcohol while taking steroids. Also, tell the doctor you are taking this drug:

- before having a vaccination

- before having any kind of surgery (including dental surgery)

- if you get a serious infection or injury

Tell your doctor if any of these or other side effects should occur:

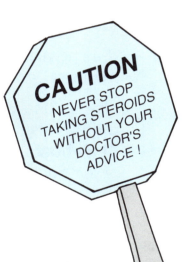

- bloody or black stools

- back or rib pain

- decreased or blurred vision

- frequent urination or increased thirst

- acne or other skin problems

- ongoing stomach pain, burning or nausea/vomiting

- unusual tiredness or weakness

- menstrual problems

- swelling of lower legs

- changes in emotions

- weight gain or redistribution of fat

- easy bruising

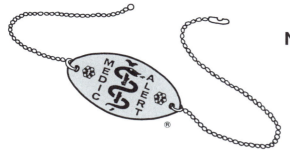

NOTE: Wear an ID bracelet or necklace (such as Medic Alert) saying you are taking steroids.

Steroid inhalers

This medicine is used to help prevent attacks of asthma. It will not help an attack once it has started. Use your steroid inhaler 20 minutes after your beta stimulator inhaler. It will take 2 to 4 weeks before the steroid inhaler will have its full effect.

Store the inhaler away from heat and direct sunlight.

Be sure to gargle and rinse your mouth after using your steroid inhaler. This may help prevent hoarseness and throat irritation. Rinsing may also help prevent thrush (Candida albicans), a fungus infection.

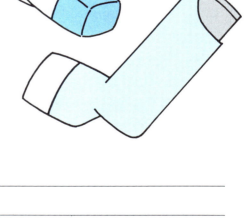

Steroid inhalers do not cause the usual side effects of steroids. But they might cause:

- hoarseness

- sore mouth or throat

- cough

Let your doctor know if any of these side effects occur.

I take:

name:_____

dose:_____

time:_____

Antibiotics

Antibiotics can be taken in the form of pills, capsules or shots. They fight bacterial infections. Take them just as your doctor tells you, and be sure to finish the entire prescription. **If you skip doses** or do not take the whole prescription, your infection can last even longer! Some of these drugs are better absorbed if you take them 30 minutes before eating and if you don't take them with milk or an antacid.

Penicillins

Penicillins are best taken on an empty stomach.

If you know you are allergic to penicillin, be sure to tell your doctor. Let your doctor know right away if any of these side effects occur:

- **hives, itching, rash, wheezing** (could mean you are allergic to penicillin)

- sore mouth or tongue

- diarrhea, nausea or vomiting

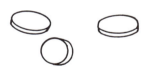

Tetracyclines

Take tetracyclines with a full glass (8 oz.) of water. If stomach upset occurs, take the medicine with food. Do not eat dairy products, drink milk or take antacids within 1 to 2 hours of the time you take tetracyclines. These will not allow the drug to work as it should. Also, do not take iron within 2 to 3 hours of the time you take tetracycline. Some people may become more sensitive to sunlight when taking this drug, so avoid too much sun.

Tetracyclines may cause these side effects:

- stomach cramps, diarrhea
- nausea, vomiting
- sore mouth or tongue
- vaginitis

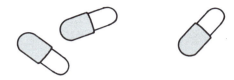

I take:

name:_____

dose:_____

time:_____

Cromolyn Sodium

This drug comes in the form of **a liquid** for use in a metered dose inhaler or **a capsule** (not used often) of powder to inhale. It is **only** for people who have allergic asthma or bronchospasm brought on by exercise. When it is inhaled regularly, it helps prevent asthma attacks, but **it is NOT to be taken during an attack.**

Possible side effects:

- throat irritation or dryness
- bad taste in the mouth
- coughing
- wheezing
- nausea
- nasal congestion

I take:

name:_____

dose:_____

time:_____

Oxygen and aerosol therapy

Oxygen

If you need it, your doctor will prescribe oxygen as one of your medicines. Treat it just like any other medicine you take. Don't change the amount unless your doctor tells you to. Oxygen should always be taken in the right amount, at the times and by the means prescribed by your doctor.

The company which provides your oxygen equipment should fully explain its use and care. When your supply arrives, be sure to find out how to reorder. Plan so that you do not run out in the middle of the night or over a weekend or holiday.

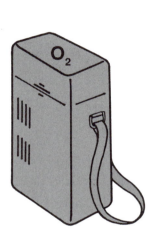

To use oxygen safely, do these:

- Store oxygen away from heat or direct sunlight.

- If using cylinders, secure them so that they cannot tip over.

- NO SMOKING in the room where oxygen is used or stored.

- Do not increase liter flow without asking your doctor.

- Do not use oxygen near an open flame (such as a gas stove or fireplace).

- You can use electric appliances. But be careful when using things that might spark (like a razor).

- Do not use any petroleum based products (such as Vaseline, certain creams, etc.).

Oxygen Company:_____ Phone #:_____

Liter Flow:_____

Hours and/or Time of Day to Use:_____

32

Aerosol therapy

There are a number of ways to spray a fine mist of medicine or moisture into your lungs. The most common ways it is done in the home are with:

- a **metered dose inhaler (MDI)**

- an **MDI with a spacer device**

- a **nebulizer**

The **metered dose inhaler** is the easiest and preferred device to use. It is a simple, portable sprayer that is mostly used for inhaling bronchodilators or steroids. Have your doctor, therapist or nurse show you the proper way to use an inhaler. There is a lot involved in its proper use.

Another way to use the MDI is with a **spacer device.** The spacer can help you coordinate the spray with your breathing. The spacer is a small tube placed between the MDI and your mouth. The medicine is sprayed into the tube and then inhaled into the lungs.

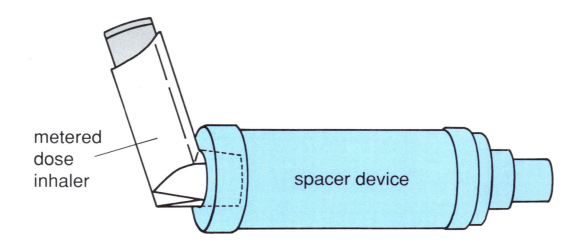

metered dose inhaler

spacer device

The **nebulizer** sprays a mist of medicine or moisture into the lungs at normal air pressure. It is mostly used for short periods several times a day.

When using a nebulizer, follow your doctor's exact instructions. Know how to use and care for your device. **If you do not clean it properly, you may give yourself a lung infection.** Your respiratory therapist, doctor and the company supplying the device will be able to teach you about its use and cleaning.

The Intermittent Positive Pressure Breathing (IPPB) machine is used only rarely. This machine carries the drug or moisture into the lungs by a flow of air under pressure. This can help you take a deeper breath.

The use of any of these devices would be prescribed by your doctor.

The following drugs should only be used on the advice of your doctor:

- **antihistamines or cold medicines** which stop your cough and dry your mucus

- **"water pills"** (diuretics) which are used to rid the body of excess fluid and can also dry your mucus

- **tranquilizers and sedatives** which relax you or help you sleep but can dangerously slow your breathing and interfere with coughing

- **narcotics** which depress breathing and stop coughing

Postural drainage

Your doctor may ask you to learn postural drainage. This is a technique that helps mucus drain out of the airways of the lungs. Be sure that you have been drinking 2 to 4 quarts of water and other fluids every day for 2 to 3 days before starting this. Mucus must be thin for postural drainage to work. If you use a bronchodilator, do postural drainage after the bronchodilator has taken effect. **Do postural drainage only when the stomach is empty.** It is best to do it first thing in the morning (1 hr. before breakfast) and in the evening (at least 1 hr. before going to bed). Your doctor or therapist will tell you:

- which positions to use

- how long to stay in each position

- how many times a day to do postural drainage

There are 4 basic postural drainage positions that help clear mucus from airways in the lower lobes of your lungs. These are:

- on your stomach

- on each side

- on your back

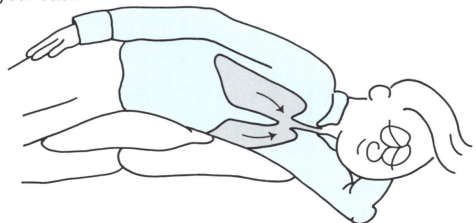

It takes about 5 to 15 minutes in each position.

Lie down in one of the 4 positions with your head and chest tilted slightly lower than the rest of your body. Lie this way, in each position, for the time your doctor has told you. Do diaphragmatic breathing (pp. 44-45) and pursed lips breathing in each position to keep airways open. Practice controlled coughing after each posture. The mucus should be easier to bring up and out. **Do not** cough in a head-down position. Always sit up to cough.

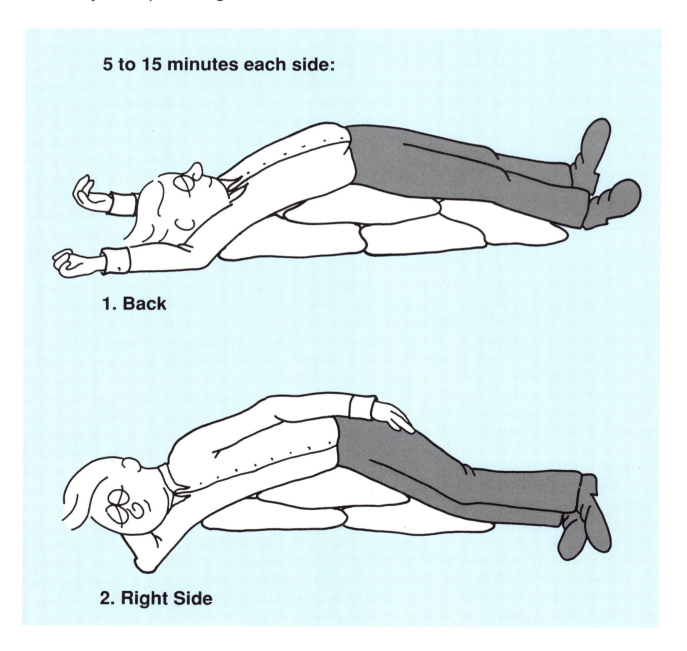

5 to 15 minutes each side:

1. Back

2. Right Side

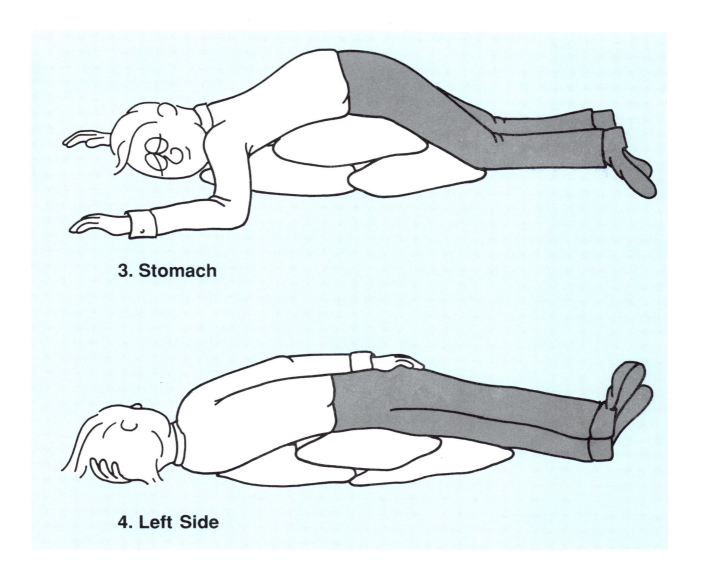

3. Stomach

4. Left Side

Your therapist or a family member may help you during postural drainage by using "cupping" and "vibration." He or she makes a "cup" with the hand and **gently thumps you on the chest or back** while you are lying in one of the positions. The thumping and percussion formed by the cupped hands loosens the trapped mucus and helps it drain. (Continue to exhale through pursed lips.) Also, cupping should be done through light clothing so it won't hurt the skin. No heavy jewelry should be worn on the hands of the person doing the cupping. Your doctor or therapist will tell you the proper amount of time and how often to use this extra help.

THUMP

Foods

This information is not for use by CF patients who must follow a very special diet. For those on a low-fat diet, avoid the foods on the next page marked with an asterisk (*).

Choose foods wisely. You need a well-balanced diet with a lot of fluids. What you eat has a direct effect on how healthy you are and how well your body is able to fight off infections. Choosing your meals from the list on the next page will help keep your body as strong and healthy as possible.

The number of servings needed from each food group every day are at the top of each list. This number of servings should be spread out over 3 small meals and 3 snacks each day.

This list will give you an idea of some amounts that equal one serving:

1/2 cup peas	1 - 6" banana
1 cup melon cubes	1 medium size potato
4 to 6 crackers	3 to 4 oz. beef
1 cup milk	1 tsp. cooking oil
1 medium fish fillet	1 oz. cheese

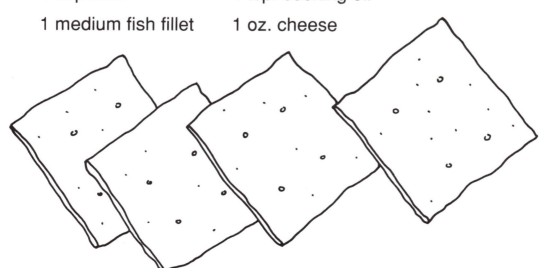

Servings to Eat Each Day
Spread out over 3 small meals and 3 snacks

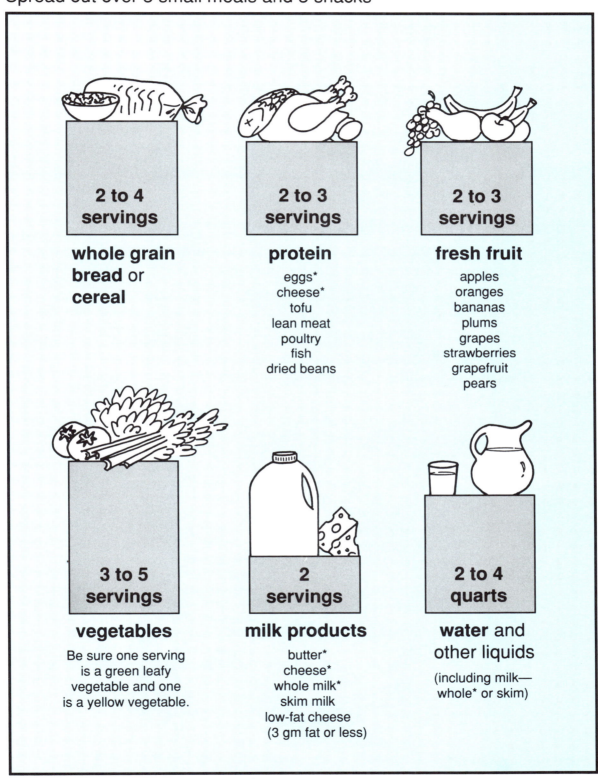

2 to 4 servings

whole grain bread or **cereal**

2 to 3 servings

protein

eggs*
cheese*
tofu
lean meat
poultry
fish
dried beans

2 to 3 servings

fresh fruit

apples
oranges
bananas
plums
grapes
strawberries
grapefruit
pears

3 to 5 servings

vegetables

Be sure one serving is a green leafy vegetable and one is a yellow vegetable.

2 servings

milk products

butter*
cheese*
whole milk*
skim milk
low-fat cheese
(3 gm fat or less)

2 to 4 quarts

water and **other liquids**

(including milk—whole* or skim)

* high in fat and/or cholestrol

If you are too thin and need to gain weight, the quickest way to add calories (without sugar or bulk) is to eat more foods with fat. Foods high in fat include:

butter	ice cream
margarine	peanut butter
vegetable oils	whole milk
red meats	milk shakes
fried foods	

If you can't eat foods with fat because of a problem with cholesterol or atherosclerosis, you can do something else. You can gain weight by eating larger amounts and not skipping meals. Another way to add calories is with diet supplements.

People with COPD should avoid a lot of sweets and desserts. These produce more carbon dioxide than other foods. The lungs have to work harder to get rid of the excess carbon dioxide.

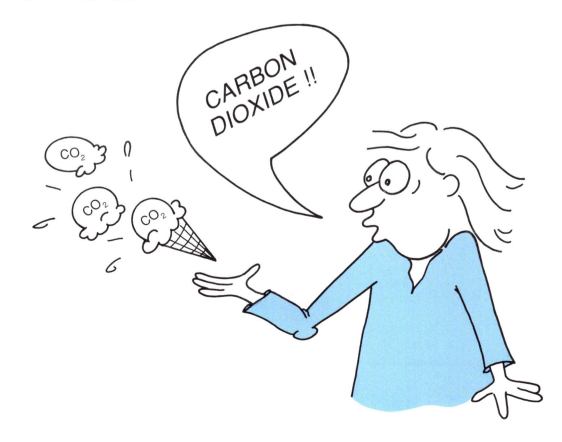

How much you eat at a time can also affect breathing. Eating a large meal can leave you feeling too full and short of breath. Eating 3 smaller meals and 3 snacks each day will make the stomach less full. This leaves more room for your lungs to expand when you breathe. Another way to avoid that "too full" feeling is to eat less of the foods that cause gas. If the foods on this list bother you, eat less of them.

apples (raw)	cucumbers
asparagas	melons
beans (pinto, kidney, black, navy)	onions (raw)
	peas (split, blackeye)
broccoli	peppers
brussels sprouts	pimientos
cabbage	radishes
carbonated drinks	rutabagas
cauliflower	turnips
corn	

WHEW

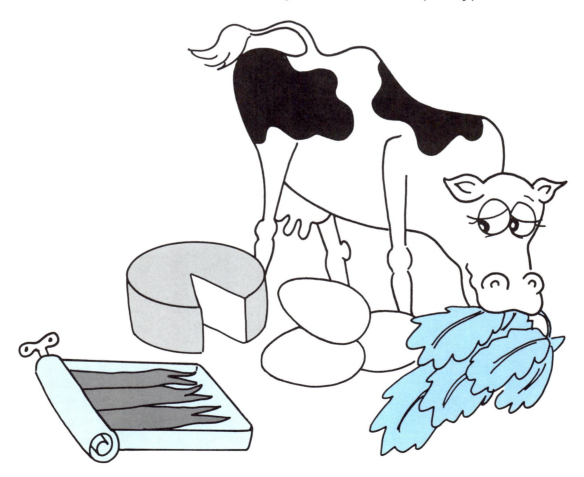

There may be days when you feel very congested with mucus. On these days, highly acid drinks like **lemonade, orange juice** or **diet cola** may help control the mucus in your throat.

Some people with COPD think that drinking milk causes increased mucus or breathing trouble. Milk does not make mucus thicker. But it may coat the back of the throat and make it feel thicker. Rinsing the mouth with water after drinking milk will prevent this problem.

If you don't drink milk, you can get calcium and protein by eating cheese, sardines with bones, green leafy vegetables, margarine, eggs and meat. Some antacids (like Tums or Rolaids) are a high source of calcium. Ask your doctor what kind and how much extra calcium you should take (if any).

Exercise

Do some exercise each day. Start out by building strength in your breathing muscles. This means your diaphragm and stomach muscles.

   In COPD the diaphragm flattens out. It doesn't do its normal share of the work of breathing. Then the work is done by the muscles around the rib cage and in the neck and shoulders. To strengthen the diaphragm, practice **diaphragmatic breathing** along with pursed lips breathing. You might also include in your daily routine other exercises which strengthen the diaphragm and the muscles in your stomach.

   Do these exercises slowly. **Don't strain.** By learning diaphragmatic and pursed lips breathing and doing other exercises to make your body strong, you will breathe better and feel better. **Think of yourself as an active person who knows how to exercise for easy breathing.** Ask your doctor or respiratory therapist which exercises are best for you.

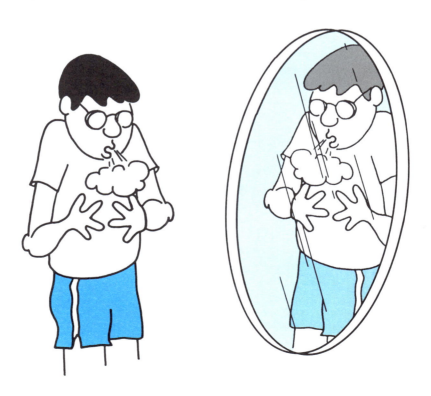

Diaphragmatic breathing

Check how the diaphragm works in these two ways:

- feel it move on the front of your abdomen

- feel it move on the sides of your abdomen

Exercise 1: Front

1. **Sit comfortably** with good posture or **lie on your back** with your head and knees supported by pillows.

2. Place one hand on your chest to check for movement of the rib cage muscles.

3. Place the other hand in the middle of your stomach to feel movement of the diaphragm.

4. Pull your stomach muscles in as you exhale slowly through pursed lips.

5. Inhale through your nose, feeling your stomach relax and **move out to the front.**

6. Rest after 3 or 4 breaths.

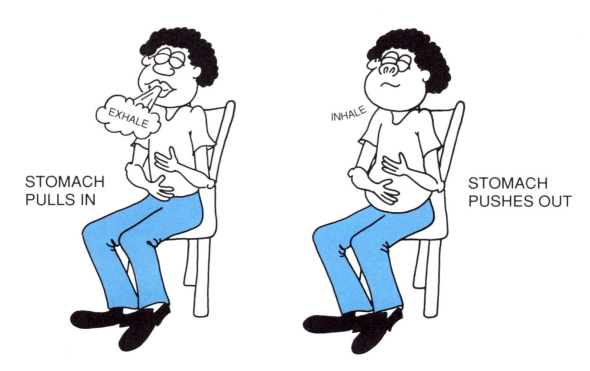

STOMACH PULLS IN

STOMACH PUSHES OUT

Exercise 2: Side

1. Sit or stand comfortably with good posture.

2. Place your hands on your sides over your lower ribs.

3. Feel your lower ribs move in as you exhale slowly through pursed lips.

4. Inhale slowly through your nose, feeling your lower ribs expand.

5. Rest after 3 or 4 breaths.

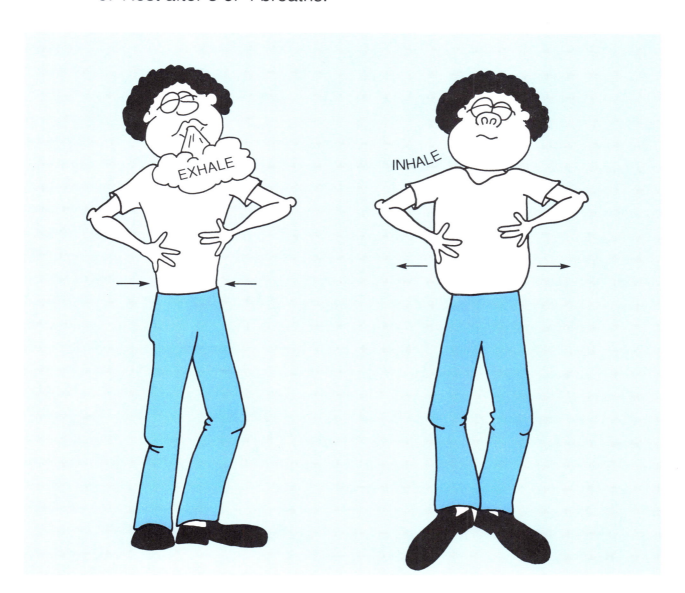

To begin with, practice both exercises 2 or 3 times a day. When you learn to do these 2 exercises well, you can make diaphragmatic breathing your normal way of breathing.

Whenever you exercise or work around the house, use diaphragmatic and pursed lips breathing. **Exhale while you do the "work" part of an exercise.** For example, exhale during a sit-up; inhale while lying back down. If you are climbing stairs, exhale as you step up and pause to inhale.

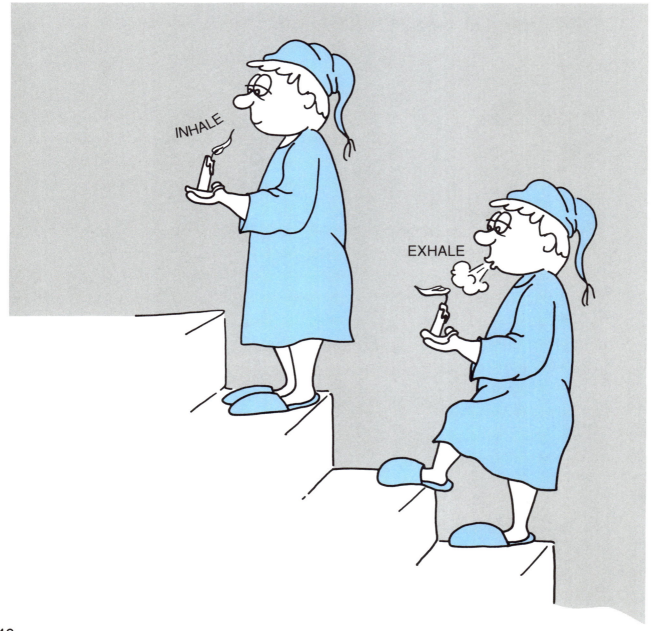

Breathing retraining exercises

These exercises help you breathe by building strength in your stomach muscles. Practice them each day. Do not do them when you feel sick or short of breath. Ask your doctor if these are OK for you.

Butterfly

1. Sit on a chair with arms at sides and feet flat on the floor.

2. Place hands behind your head and raise arms shoulder high, breathing slowly through the nose.

3. As you breathe out slowly through pursed lips, slowly bend over towards your knees, bringing elbows in toward your face. Bend over only as far as is comfortable.

4. Inhale as you slowly return to a sitting position.

5. Rest.

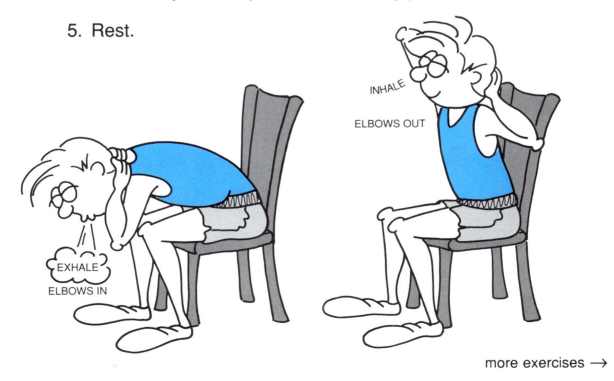

EXHALE
ELBOWS IN

INHALE
ELBOWS OUT

more exercises →

Knee to chest

1. Lie **flat on your back*** on floor with knees bent and feet flat on the floor.

2. Inhale slowly through nose.

3. Bring right knee to chest as you slowly exhale through pursed lips.

4. Pull knee tightly towards chest with hands.

5. Slowly lower right foot to the floor, as you inhale through your nose.

6. Rest.

7. Repeat with your left leg.

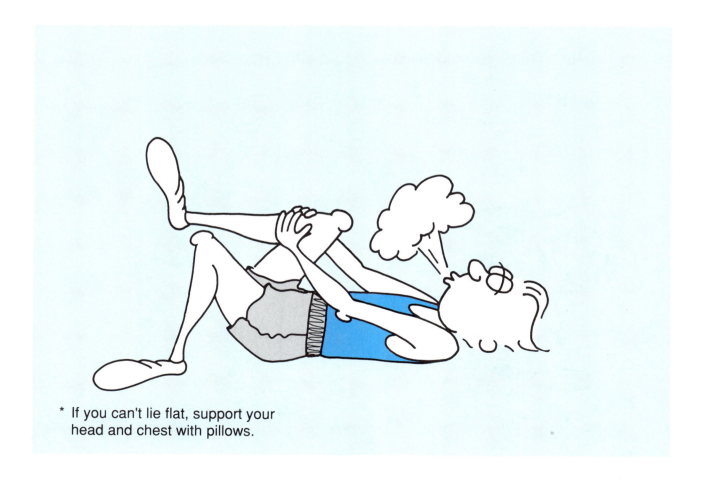

* If you can't lie flat, support your head and chest with pillows.

Partial sit-ups

1. Lie **flat on your back*** on the floor with knees bent and arms at sides.

2. Sit up toward your knees, raising shoulders only about 8 inches off the floor, as you exhale through pursed lips. Arms should extend beside knees, but don't hold on.

3. Lower yourself to floor as you inhale through nose.

   Be sure not to use your neck muscles to sit up. Use your stomach (abdominal) muscles. This exercise is to strengthen the stomach muscles.

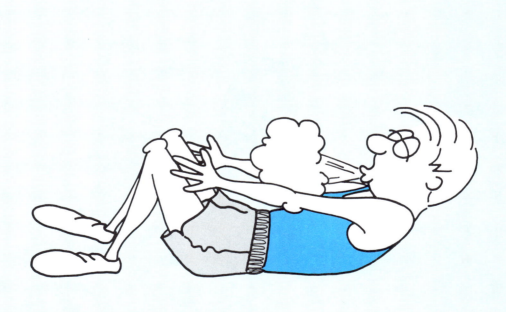

* If you can't lie flat, support your head and chest with pillows.

Other exercise

Walking and riding a stationary bike are also good exercises for people with COPD. Before you walk or ride:

- practice pursed lips breathing

- do breathing retraining exercises

- do stretching exercises (see next page)

Find out if there is a pulmonary rehabilitation program in your community hospital. They can test you and find out the safest exercise for you. Medicare and many private insurance companies will cover all or part of the costs for pulmonary rehab.

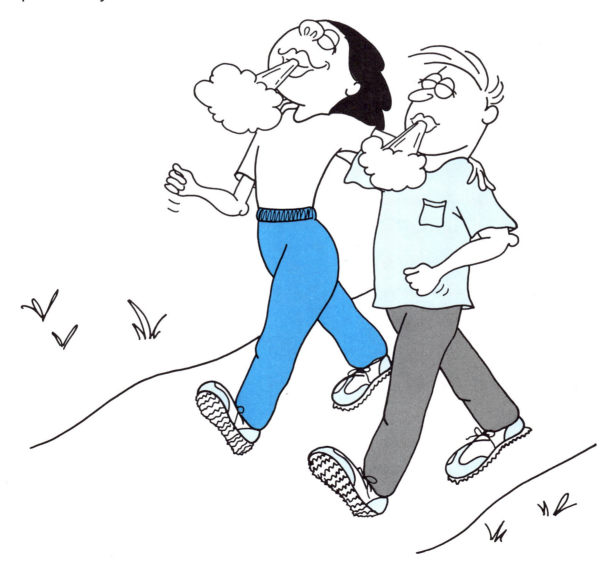

Stretching, warm-up, cool-down

Stretching exercises will help loosen the muscles in your neck, shoulders and chest which your breathing problems cause to get tight and sore. Here is an example of a good stretch for people with lung disease.

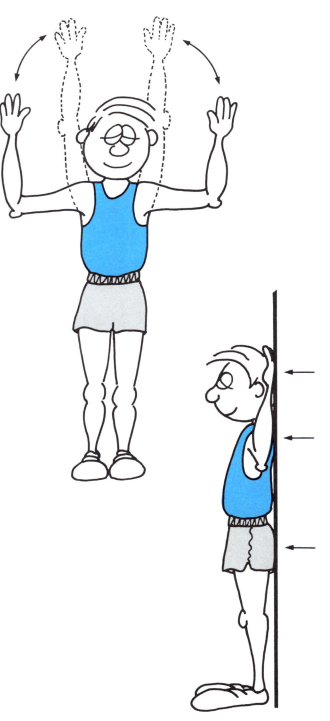

1. Stand with your back against the wall. Shoulders and bottom touch the wall. Heels are 3 inches from wall.

2. Bring your arms out to the side with elbows bent so that both arms rest against the wall.

3. Slowly slide your arms overhead as you straighten your elbows and inhale. **Keep your arms, elbows and bottom in touch with the wall** as you slide your arms overhead. (At first you may only be able to stretch them part of the way.)

4. Slide your arms down to the starting position as you exhale.

5. Repeat 3 - 5 times.

Sex

Having a chronic health problem can upset any relationship for awhile, and this includes sex. But don't write off sex as something you can't enjoy because you have COPD. It is likely that you can function better sexually than you believe.

Start by talking with your partner. Roles and feelings have probably changed as you and your partner got used to your lung condition. Sharing how each of you feels can renew your relationship and sex life. As you talk, it may help to remember these:

- You are still a sexual being with needs and desires.

- Human sexual response is not confined to the sex organs or to orgasm.

- You can show affection by hugging, kissing and touching each other.

- Giving and receiving are not always equal in a relationship.

- It is hard to be sexy if you are anxious, depressed or bothered by guilt, old habits or anger.

- Anxiety can increase shortness of breath during sex.

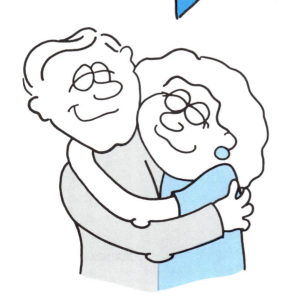

You may face other problems as well. Your partner may fear that sex will be too hard on your breathing. Less oxygen in your blood may cause you to feel restless and touchy. These problems can be solved by time and by talking openly with your partner. Not talking about them will only increase the tension, doubts, anger or frustration that either of you have.

As a person gets older, there are some changes that occur. (This is true whether the person has a chronic illness or not.) Some of these changes are:

- It takes more time for orgasm to occur.

- There may be a decrease in vaginal lubrication.

- It may take longer to have an erection following ejaculation.

- Some medicines may cause a change in sexual function.

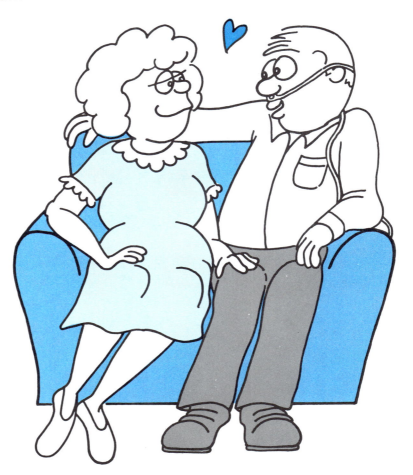

Your body during sex

Think about the changes your body goes through during sex. The skin becomes flushed. Your heartbeat and breathing rate increase. As you reach orgasm, which lasts about 15 to 20 seconds, your heart may beat as often as 130-150 times per minute. Your breathing will be fast. Then, within seconds, your body returns to normal. (You can use pursed lips breathing to help slow your breathing.) These are normal body changes during sex and are not harmful to you even if you have trouble breathing. Be sure and allow plenty of time for sexual foreplay. This gives your body time to adjust to the changes that occur.

Above all, keep up your daily breathing and exercise program. A strong body can handle sex better and will help you feel better about yourself and sex.

Just keep in mind:

- relax
- slow down
- enjoy each other

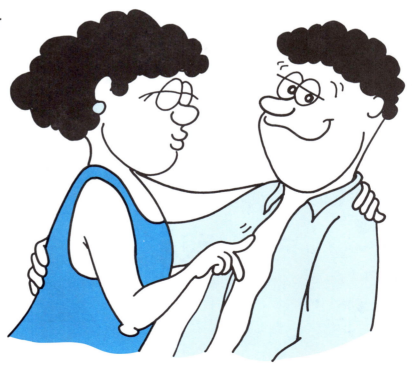

Better breathing during sex

These may help you to breathe more easily during sex:

- Choose the best time of day for breathing, and be rested.

- Always wait 2 to 3 hours after a meal.

- Keep the room cool.

- **Plan to have sex after your bronchodilator has taken effect.**

- If you use oxygen daily, nasal prongs worn during sex will not interfere with sex.

- Don't rush. Give yourself plenty of time to engage in foreplay in a relaxed atmosphere.

- If you start to get anxious, STOP. Relax, cuddle.

- **Make pleasure and affection your goal,** whether you reach orgasm or not.

Try new positions. Find the ones most comfortable for you and your partner. Avoid positions which make you support your body on your arms or put added pressure on your stomach. Since you breathe better with your head and chest elevated, you might try these positions:

- side-lying, either face to face or male behind female

- female on top — male can recline against the headboard or sit in a chair

- female sitting with male kneeling or standing

Both partners must share in meeting each other's physical and emotional needs. Talking with your partner and using what you have learned can speed you both on your way to a better sex life.

When to call your doctor

You need to know the first signs of an infection or respiratory problem that call for immediate treatment. Discuss these symptoms with your doctor. He or she may want you to get in touch at once when one or more of these occur.

- more shortness of breath, difficulty in breathing or wheezing than usual

- more coughing (more often, more severe or both)

- increase or decrease in mucus production

- change in color of mucus (to yellow, grey, green or bloody)

- swelling in ankles, legs, around eyes

- sudden weight gain (3-5 pounds overnight)

- heart palpitations or faster pulse than usual

- unusual dizziness, sleepiness, headaches, vision problems, irritability, trouble thinking

- loss of appetite (more than usual)

- dehydration (shown by concentrated urine and dry skin)

- fever

- early morning headaches not relieved by mild headache medicines (such as aspirin, Tylenol, etc.)

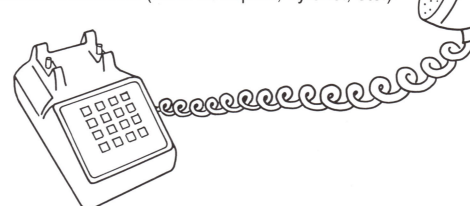

Checklist for PART 2

Check the things you use to control your lung problem.

☐ To control wheezing, I use pursed lips breathing, take my prescribed bronchodilator and drink plenty of fluids.

☐ I do not smoke.

☐ I do my best to avoid things that can make my problem worse: air pollution, very cold air, air that is too humid (or too dry), strong fumes, dust and things I am allergic to.

☐ I have accepted the fact that I have a lung disease and am using a positive attitude about treatment. I talk my fears or depression out with those who can help me.

☐ I use relaxation exercises to relieve muscle tension and anxiety.

☐ I take my medicine(s) just as they are prescribed. The medicine(s) I take are:

_____ (p.___)

_____ (p.___)

_____ (p.___)

☐ I know how to use my inhaler properly.

☐ I use postural drainage (if prescribed).

☐ I eat a well-balanced diet with a lot of fluids.

☐ I do diaphragmatic breathing every day.

continued on next page

☐ I do breathing retraining exercises every day.

☐ I do some exercise each day.

☐ I do stretches each day.

☐ My partner and I share our feelings about my lung disease and work together to make our relationship a warm and satisfying one for both of us.

☐ I know the signs of infection and to call my doctor should they occur.

Notes: _____

_____

_____

_____

_____

_____

_____

_____

_____

_____

_____

_____

_____

_____

_____

_____

_____

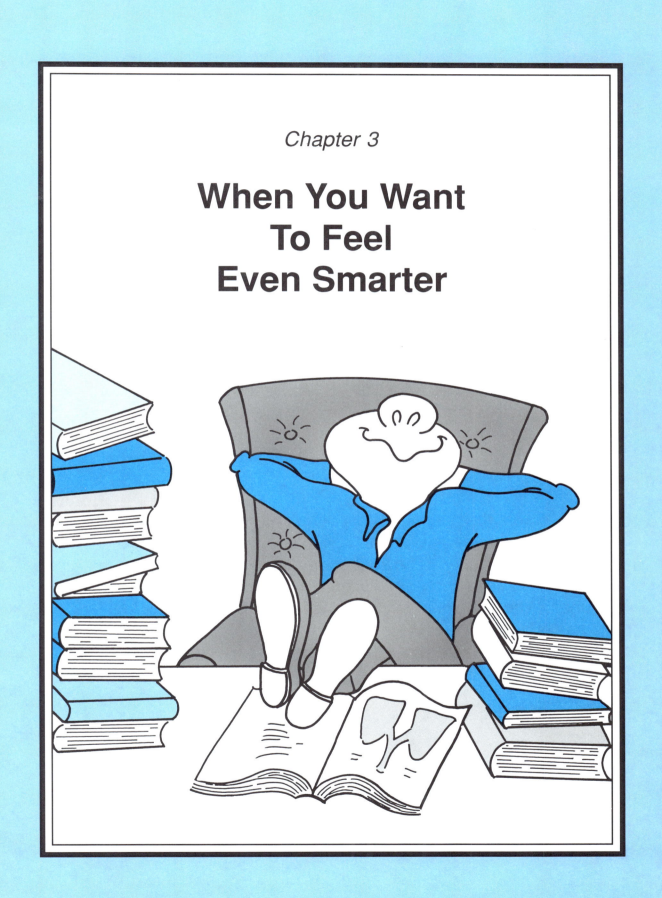

Chapter 3

When You Want
To Feel
Even Smarter

Normal lungs and normal breathing

Each breath you take in gives your body the oxygen it needs to live. Each time you exhale, the body gets rid of carbon dioxide which it produces as waste. The lungs remove carbon dioxide from the blood so you can exhale it.

If your air supply were cut off for about 5 minutes, your body would run out of the oxygen it needs. And if you couldn't exhale the carbon dioxide your body makes, the buildup in your blood would soon cause headaches, fatigue and drowsiness.

Most of the work to get air in and out of the lungs is done by the **diaphragm.** This is a sheet of muscle that separates your chest from your stomach cavity **(abdomen).** Your lungs are sealed in an airtight cavity. When your diaphragm moves down, this airtight cavity expands. This creates a vacuum which sucks air into the lungs. When the diaphragm relaxes, it lets air flow back out of the lungs.

Air enters the body through your mouth or nose. The mouth and nose clean the air and bring it to the right wetness and body temperature. The air then enters the windpipe **(trachea)** and flows through two large air tubes **(bronchi)** to the lungs. The right lung has three parts or **lobes,** and the left lung has two.

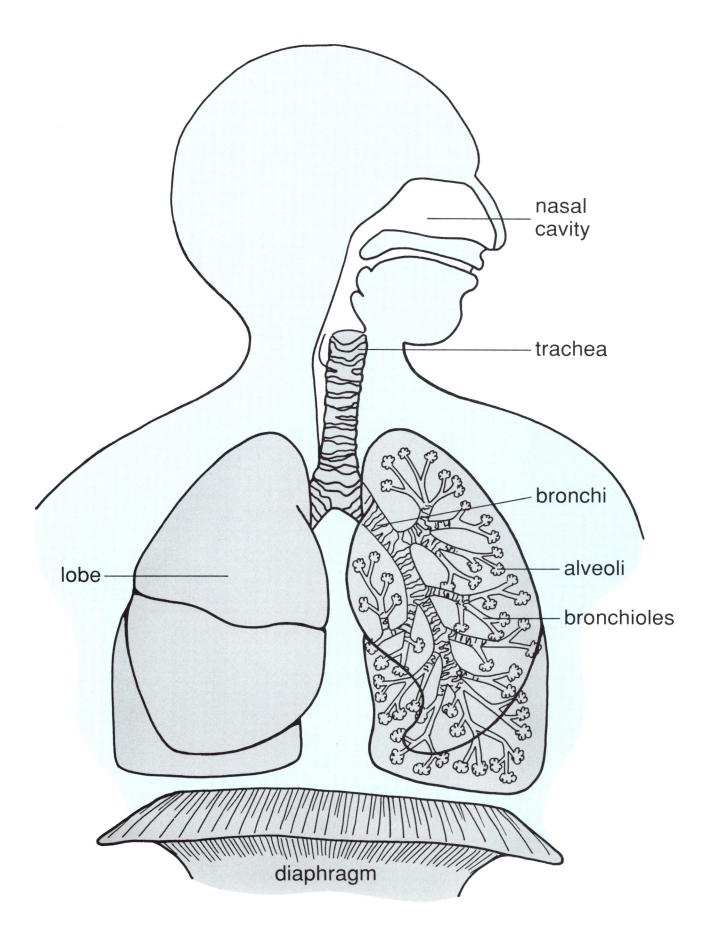

nasal
cavity

trachea

bronchi

alveoli

bronchioles

lobe

diaphragm

61

The bronchi supply all parts of the lungs with air by splitting again and again into smaller bronchi which run through all five lobes of the lungs. The bronchi divide into even smaller air tubes **(bronchioles)** and end finally in 300 million tiny, elastic air sacs **(alveoli).**

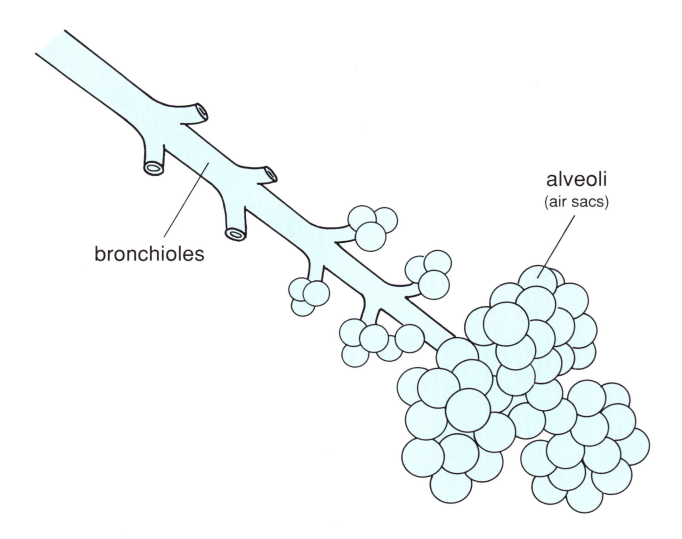

bronchioles

alveoli
(air sacs)

If the air which enters the lungs still contains gases or dirt, the airways in the lungs have a system to clean it. All breathing tubes are lined with mucus and cells which have tiny hairs **(cilia).** Other cells in the airways make mucus which lies on top of the cilia. There are millions of cilia, all sweeping mucus toward the mouth. Inhaled dirt is trapped on the mucus and is pushed up the windpipe, where it is swallowed or coughed out. So by the time oxygen reaches the alveoli, it is clean and ready to be picked up by the blood and carried to all parts of the body.

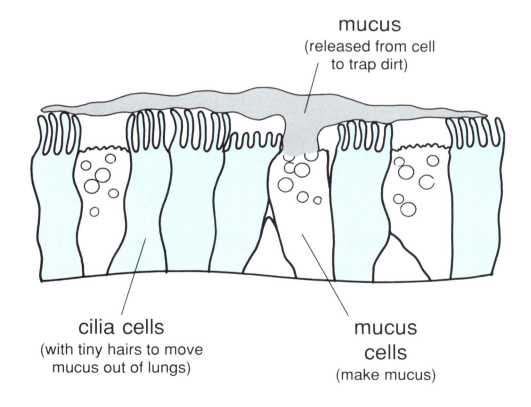

mucus
(released from cell
to trap dirt)

cilia cells
(with tiny hairs to move
mucus out of lungs)

mucus
cells
(make mucus)

The walls of the alveoli are about as thick as a soap bubble just before it bursts. Running through these walls are tiny blood tubes **(capillaries).** Your lungs have about 3 billion capillaries. Oxygen easily passes into these tiny blood tubes from the air sacs. And carbon dioxide crosses into the air sacs where it is left to be exhaled.

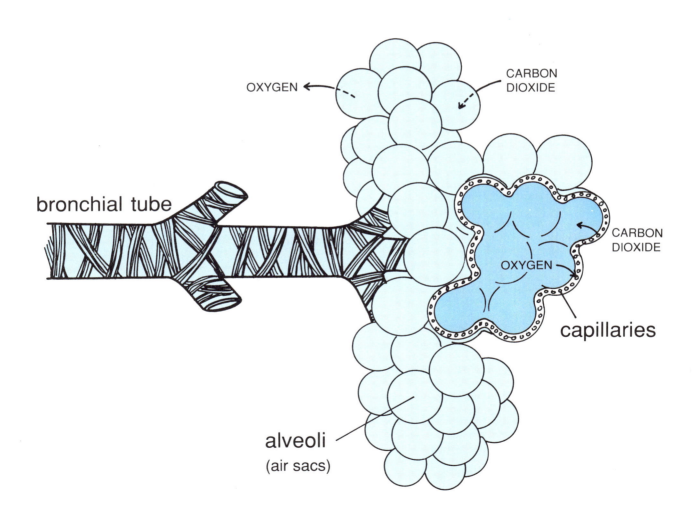

Chronic bronchitis

Chronic bronchitis is brought on by:

- cigarette smoke

- air pollution

- allergens

Any of these may bother the lining of the bronchial tubes so much that the lining swells and makes excess mucus. It becomes harder to breathe, and a chronic cough and wheezing develop as a result of this mucus. Some air tubes may even be blocked by excess mucus. When this happens, you are more likely to have lung infections which may do lasting damage to the lungs.

normal
bronchial tube
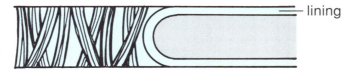

chronic
bronchitis
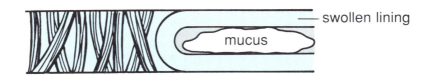

Antibiotics can cure bacterial infections, but they can't cure chronic bronchitis itself. The best way to stop the progress of chronic bronchitis is:

- **avoid the irritant causing the disease (especially cigarette smoke)**

- drink a lot of fluids

- keep your lungs cleared of mucus

- use postural drainage

- take medicines prescribed for you

Emphysema

Emphysema is a disease of the air sacs, though it causes airway blockage too. Most emphysema is caused by cigarette smoke. The air sacs, blood vessels and support tissue are destroyed. Many of the small air tubes collapse. With emphysema, this happens:

- The transfer of oxygen and carbon dioxide is impaired. (Lung reserve capacity is decreased.)

- Extra pressure is needed to exhale; some small and even some large airways (bronchial tubes) may collapse.

- The body has to work harder to get air out.

- More mucus is trapped in the lungs, making them prone to infection.

- Shortness of breath and coughing increase.

- Over time, the lungs and even the heart may become enlarged.

Emphysema has no cure, though medications and breathing exercises (including pursed lips breathing) help. **Not smoking** and avoiding other irritants will help slow the progress of the disease.

Most people with COPD have both emphysema and bronchitis.

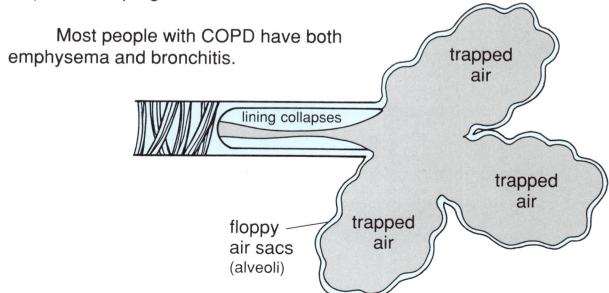

trapped air

lining collapses

trapped air

floppy air sacs (alveoli)

trapped air

Asthma

If you have asthma, your airways are much more sensitive than normal. You may have allergies to such things as:

- pollen

- animals

- dust

- aspirin

Your airways may react to hard exercise, infections, cold air or polluted air.

When you inhale irritants, the linings of the bronchioles in your lungs swell and make excess mucus. The muscles in the walls of these airways go into spasm and clamp down on the airways. You wheeze and feel short of breath.

Most often the treatment for asthma is:

- avoid the cause

- take bronchodilator drugs

- drink lots of fluids

- practice controlled coughing and pursed lips breathing

- do postural drainage (not during an acute attack)

bronchial muscles spasm

The drugs relax the muscles in the airways and make it easier to breathe. Using pursed lips breathing and coughing up mucus during an asthma attack can help open up your airways.

Bronchiectasis

Bronchiectasis can be caused by:

- a serious lung infection, often in early childhood

- abnormal lung development before birth
  or during childhood

It is common in children who have cystic fibrosis. In bronchiectasis, scar tissue which makes too much mucus replaces the walls of the airways. The airways deep in the lungs become widened sacs where mucus can pool. The mucous membrane and bronchial muscles are not able to push this pooled mucus up to the throat to be expelled. So you may cough, wheeze and suffer from shortness of breath and excess mucus. Another problem may be persistent infection of the mucus.

Treatment includes water drinking, postural drainage, antibiotics, pursed lips breathing and bronchodilators.

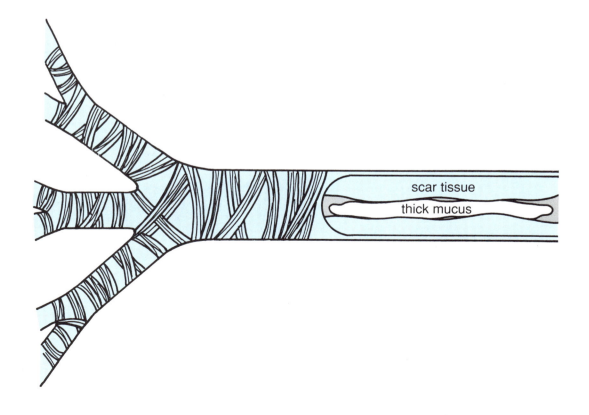

scar tissue

thick mucus

Cystic fibrosis

Cystic fibrosis (CF) affects the lungs and the digestive system. People with CF are born with it though it sometimes does not show up until later. They inherit the disease in the genes they get from both parents.

In the lungs of a CF patient, thick, sticky mucus blocks the airways. This makes breathing harder and causes coughing and wheezing. Because of these blockages, the lungs become infected easily and often. This leads to lasting damage of the alveoli, bronchioles and bronchi.

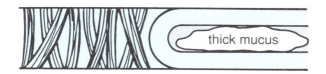

Treatment for the respiratory problems caused by CF includes using antibiotics to keep the lungs as clear of infection as possible. You can help to prevent problems by doing breathing exercises and postural drainage, drinking a lot of fluids and using aerosol therapy and bronchodilators.

CF has no cure, but with early diagnosis and use of antibiotics for lung infections, one in two people with CF will reach age 20. Many will live much longer. Continuing advances in diagnosis and treatment offer even more promise in life expectancy and quality of life for people with CF.

You can learn more about cystic fibrosis from:

Cystic Fibrosis Foundation
600 Executive Boulevard
Rockville, MD 20852

(301) 881-9130 or
1-800-FIGHT CF

Checklist for PART 3

My chronic lung problem is:_____

Things to remember (refer to the one(s) relating to you):

- Chronic bronchitis is brought on by: cigarette smoke, air pollution, allergens. (See p. 65.)

- Most emphysema is caused by cigarette smoking. (See p. 66.)

- Asthma can be caused by allergies, reaction to hard exercise, infections, cold air or polluted air. (See p. 67.)

- Bronchiectasis can be caused by a serious infection or abnormal lung development. (See p. 68.)

- Cystic fibrosis affects the lungs and the digestive system. (See p. 69.)

Notes:_____
_____
_____
_____
_____
_____
_____
_____

Questions (for my doctor, nurse, therapist):_____
_____
_____
_____
_____
_____

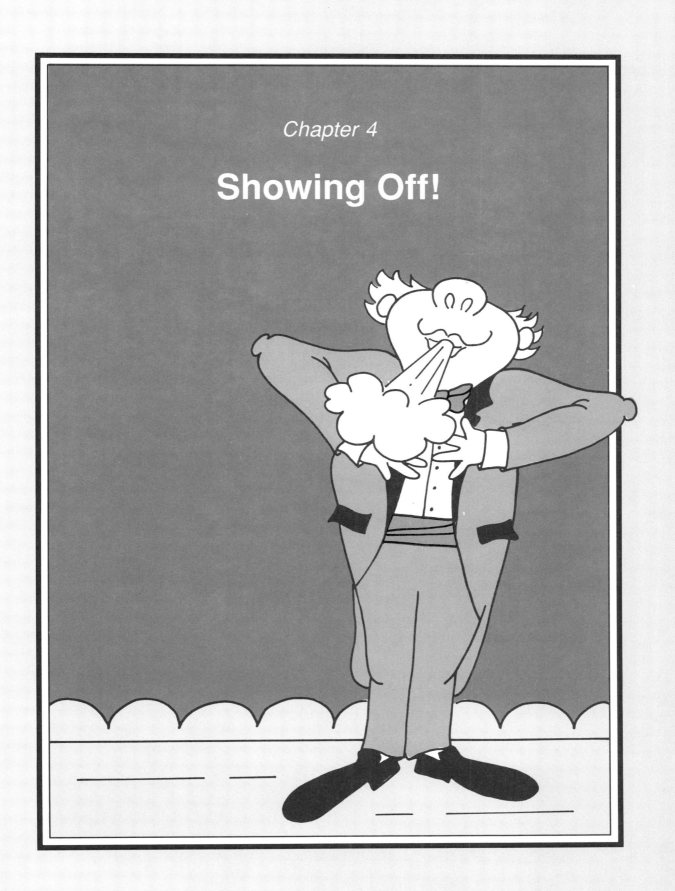

Chapter 4

Showing Off!

When you know as much about your lungs and lung disease as you do now, why not show off? Put to work what you have learned in this book and from other sources, and stick to your treatment each day. While taking care of your lungs, do these:

- Ask your doctor, nurse or respiratory therapist any questions you may have.

- Drink lots of fluids each day (unless not allowed for other health reasons).

- Use the drugs prescribed for you.

- Make breathing and body exercises a daily habit.

- Practice postural drainage (if told to do so by your doctor).

- Eat foods that will keep you healthy and help you fight infection.

- Talk with your family about the changes made in your life by COPD.

- Choose a goal and work toward reaching it.

Show off. Work a little magic on your lung disease, and breathe as easily as you can.

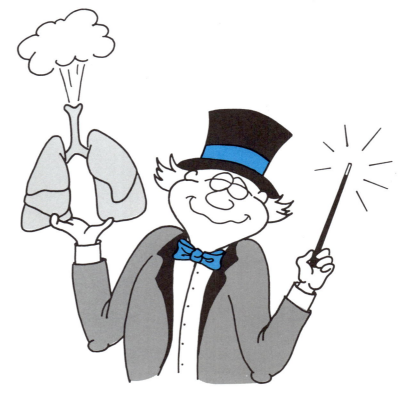